Find your iKiGAi

Find your iKiGAi

Suzanne H Visser

C_P^M

CONTENTS

Note! What follows is not medical advice.

If you need medical advice, see a doctor or consider consulting a psychiatrist or psychologist.

Welcome to this guide. It arose from a combination of personal experience and research and is designed to help you to enhance your well-being in a gentle, supportive manner. The content and order are organised in a sequence, but it's completely flexible, so feel free to move through it at whatever pace and order feels comfortable. You're the best judge of your own body and mind, so go easy and pay attention to what resonates.

The book begins with background information on *ikigai* and flow. From there, it transitions into a series of somatic practices, suggested over a period of eleven weeks. These are easy, body-focused activities designed to reset your nervous system and promote a sense of safety. This weekly structure is just a guideline; you might spend more or less time on any part, repeating as needed or skipping ahead if something doesn't quite fit right now. After the practices, the book continues with more thoughts on discovering meaning, maintaining health, and personal growth.

If certain activities feel challenging due to physical limitations, health concerns, or other reasons, the appendix provides adaptations to make them more accessible.

It is essential to set aside any self-judgment throughout your time with these practices.

For those who are older, are in pain, experienced burnout, or were traumatised

The Number 1 to Well-Being

I have a friend who is in his mid-seventies, disabled by an illness, and in a lot of pain, both physically and mentally. He likes reading, but his days often consist of waiting for bedtime. He rarely experiences a sense of fulfilment or meaning. He isolates himself. He often feels frozen and anxious. Let's call him Peter.

I have another friend who is of the same age, much more disabled than Peter, often in a lot of pain physically, but okay mentally. He enjoys life, has a lot of friends and is relaxed and joyful. Let's call him Oliver.

Both have no religion or follow any other spiritual path. In knowing and observing them both, I learn about the difference between pain and suffering. Peter clearly suffers. Oliver has pain but is not suffering.

Although Oliver is much more disabled than Peter, he is thriving, and Peter is withering. Why is this? It is this difference that interests me. The difference between Peter and Oliver can be explained through ikigai, a Japanese concept that is often translated as meaning. Not the meaning of life in general (the meaning people often find in religion or spirituality), but a sense of personal meaning. Peter does not have much of such a sense; Oliver does. Peter does not often experience ikigai, a reason to get up in the morning; Oliver does.

In older age, the importance of ikigai becomes increasingly evident.

I know someone who was a nurse his entire working life and who has the same disability as Peter. He is the same age as Peter. Let's call him Michael. He is cheerful and physically active. This is not easy for him, but he knows from experience that it is vital. Michael told me of his general observation as a nurse of those who have much better outcomes than others:

1. They have a strong social network (doctors, nurses, carers, helpers, friends, family, community)
2. They have a positive attitude. They do not complain. They take full responsibility for their condition. They display curiosity towards their condition and research it. They look for solutions and better outcomes outside the medical system (diet, movement, socialising, a method for coping, for example, Stoicism or meditation)
3. They move. Whatever small capacity they have, they move the body parts that they can move, even when in pain
4. Only after these four points are taken care of do they seek medical intervention
5. They research better diets, if needed with the help of a dietician. For example, they switch to vegetarian, plant-based, and/ or organic food

In that very order.

Even if points 2 to 5 are not engaged in, patients who engage in point 1 do much better than others. I double-checked this with my uncle, a retired surgeon in his eighties who still works occasionally. He confirms: those who show up and participate, even if they are old, disabled or in pain, do much better in all fields than those who isolate. Even those who have a pet do better than those who don't.

Research, too numerous to mention, shows that connection to others is the number one key to human well-being.

2

Attention and Meaning

Meaning can come from many places: from the people we love, the animals who share our lives, the work we do, the places we visit, and the experiences that stay with us. For some, it may be found in art or learning. For others, it might arise from caring for family, being part of a club or community, or enjoying quiet moments. Meaning is different for everyone, shaped by personal history, values and circumstances.

Attention plays a central role in how meaning forms. It influences what we notice and what we overlook, what we nurture and what we allow to fade. The sense of meaning lives not only in the thing, person or experience itself, but in the way we engage with it.

Imagine your home is on fire. Everyone you love, including pets, is already safe. You have time to take just a handful of things. What would you choose? In a way, we are always in that burning house. Life presents us with similar choices every day: what to give our energy to, what to keep close, and what to let go of.

Ikigai is that feeling of meaningfulness. It is what gives life a sense of worth. It is what makes a person want to get up in the morning.

When we lose our sense of meaning, the effects can touch every part of life. We feel empty, hopeless or disconnected. Motivation fades, and it can be challenging to take pleasure in activities that once mattered. We may withdraw from others or reduce participation in work and hobbies. A loss of meaning is linked to poorer health outcomes, such as reduced immunity, higher inflammation and shorter life expectancy. Our identity can also be shaken, especially if meaning was tied to a role or activity that is no longer part of our lives. Without a clear sense of meaning, decisions may feel aimless or paralysing. Even when opportunities appear, they may be passed by because nothing seems worth pursuing.

Recovery from this condition begins with very small steps, such as reconnecting with supportive relationships, engaging in activities that evoke curiosity or enjoyment, and re-establishing daily routines that nurture health and stability. Sometimes professional support is helpful, particularly when the loss of meaning is accompanied by persistent low mood.

Ikigai is a feeling (kan) that can be rebuilt. Even when it fades, it can return through consistent, gentle attention to what matters.

I invite you to reflect on what matters most to you. Dedicate an hour to this, more if you want. Use a digital notebook if the page isn't enough or you don't want to write.

What matters most to me

I lost meaning because

Meaning I can find right now

Social

Community

Body

Activity

Relaxation

Burdens that need to be put down

Example:

I lost meaning because
I am getting old. I'm losing mobility and energy. My family have
moved on.

Meaning I can find right now

Social
My friends mean a lot to me. I have been reconnecting to them. I
do an effort to meet for coffee and conversation.

Community
I run a community board on Facebook.

Body
I reconnect with my body through exercise. I know I feel better
when I do. I jump (rebound) on a small trampoline and do reformer
Pilates. I pay attention to balance. I take baths and do toe exercises
and somatic work while in it.
I have cut out sugar and make everything from scratch. I buy organic fruit and veg.

Activity
I am a publisher and writer. Soon I will have a PhD, a Dr title.
Do I really want to become a legal consultant? Or should I remain in
academia? I better find someone to talk with about this. My supervi-
sor seems th right place to start.

Relaxation

I like watching movies.

Burdens that need to be put down
I need to get rid of more stuff I own (just a little).
The end of self-improvement is here.
The end of buying things is here. (I can go to lawn sales to experience retail therapy if I must).
Should I sell my car and start cycling?

When I Lost My Ikigai

I tried again to swing my legs over the edge of the bed. It should have been a simple movement, but each attempt ended the same way: I collapsed back onto the mattress in pain, my legs refusing to cooperate. My spine felt as though it had given way, and I felt the same. I had just finished my PhD thesis.

I was a legal consultant, a Japanese calligraphy practitioner, a body-work coach, an artist, an HR specialist, a mother, a grand-mother, a publisher, a traveller, a sustainable justice scholar, a managing director, and someone who loved coffee, matcha and flowers, but what did these things still mean now that I could not move?

Soon, I would need to get up to use the toilet. The thought made me groan aloud. This was not the first time my back had failed me, but the pain was worse than ever before, a relentless fire in my lower spine. An MRI once again showed nothing to explain it. My back pain had always been "unexplained". I knew that the real cause was complex. Somewhere along the way, I had lost my ikigai. I knew, although it was completely counterintuitive, that I had to move. I had to get myself to the yoga mat that was about six meters away. It took me hours, but I went to the yoga mat and began the practices described in this book. Then, I called a friend to discuss my condition with.

I had once felt it vividly, in the calm focus of calligraphy, in the simple joy of being absorbed in a task. But years of ambition, responsibility and pushing through warning signs had smothered that feeling. My life was full of achievements, but the thread that made them feel alive had gone missing.

How does someone lose their ikigai? It can slip away gradually, buried under the weight of obligations and unrelieved stress, or vanish suddenly when health, work or relationships change. Without it, life can feel like a series of tasks without purpose. Pain is the worst culprit, but also a fierce but fantastic teacher.

The question that followed was unavoidable: how could I find my ikigai again?

This book is my attempt to answer that, to show how ikigai can be rediscovered and how, in the process, we can invite back the states of glow and flow that make life worth living.

While I'm working on this book, it is my ikigai.

The Japanese Understanding of Ikigai

Ikigai is a Japanese word that is often translated as "reason for being." In Japan, it does not usually mean one grand life purpose. It is more about the small and ordinary things that make life feel worth living.

Ikigai can come from many sources: caring for children or grandchildren, growing vegetables, walking with friends, serving customers with pride, practising a craft, being part of a local club, enjoying a morning cup of tea, listening to music, or tending to a garden.

Rather than being something to hunt for or achieve, ikigai in the Japanese sense often arises naturally from the way a person lives. It grows out of the roles they hold, the relationships they maintain, the routines they follow, and the contributions they make to family or community.

Ikigai is closely linked to other Japanese values. *Mottainai* is the sense of not wasting what is precious, whether that is food, resources, or opportunities. *Gaman* is the ability to endure hardship with patience and dignity. *Wabi-sabi* is an appreciation of simplicity and imperfection. These values shape an understanding of ikigai that is about living with attention, balance, and care.

Ikigai can change with life stages. What feels important in youth may be different in later years, but the principle remains the same: life has worth because of the things, people and experiences that bring meaning.

Iikigai is not a fixed goal or a single calling. It is a way of being that makes space for purpose and connection. It supports resilience during hard times and deepens appreciation during good times. When circumstances change, there is something to hold on to, and that something can help one rise each morning.

The Western Understanding of Ikigai

The West has given its own spin to the word *ikigai*. In the West, *ikigai* is explained through four overlapping circles. Each circle represents a key element:

1. What you love
2. What you are good at
3. What the world needs
4. What you can be paid for or otherwise valued for

Where all four circles overlap is presented as your ikigai. This version is widely used in self-help, career coaching and entrepreneurship because it offers a structured way to think about purpose.

The Western interpretation emphasises personal choice and agency. It suggests that a fulfilling life comes from identifying your passions, talents, the needs of others, and opportunities to earn a living, then bringing those elements together. It is often used to help people plan careers, start new ventures or make life changes that feel more aligned with their values.

While this model can be inspiring, it differs from the Japanese view. In Japan, ikigai is rarely tied so closely to paid work or financial reward.

The Western model can be a useful tool; however, it is only one way of thinking about ikigai. When combined with the Japanese understanding, it offers a broader perspective; one that values both practical goals and the quieter, everyday sources of meaning.

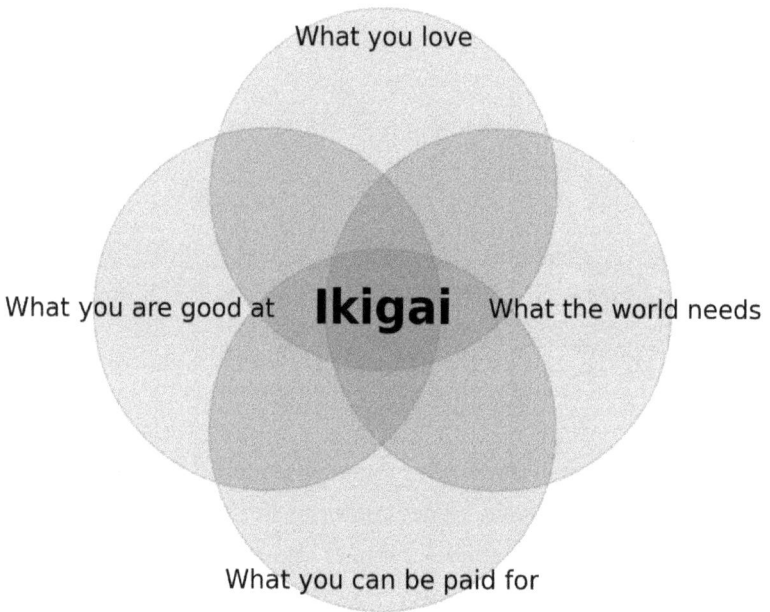

What you love

What you are good at   Ikigai   What the world needs

What you can be paid for

Good Ideas

In the West, the Ten Rules of Ikigai have become popular in books, articles and talks about living well. They are often presented as habits or attitudes that support a long and meaningful life, inspired by the lifestyles of people in Okinawa, Japan.

While these suggestions can be valuable, calling them "rules" seems not quite right. A rule implies something fixed and universal that must be followed. Ikigai is personal. It is shaped by culture, relationships, values and life stage. What works for one person may not suit another. Treating these ideas as rules can make ikigai feel like a set of instructions to complete, rather than something to discover and grow in your own way.

It seems more useful to think of them as good ideas for living with ikigai. Good ideas are flexible. They invite you to try them, adapt them and keep what fits. They leave space for your own experiences and changing needs.

They are not meant to be obeyed. They are starting points for reflection, small experiments and gentle adjustments. In this spirit, the following pages share the Ten Rules of Ikigai, reframed as ten good ideas. You may find that some are already part of your life, while others are worth exploring.

Here are the ten good ideas:

1. **Surround yourself with good friends**
Relationships bring warmth, laughter, support and perspective. Spending time with people you trust and enjoy is the strongest contributor to well-being. When you get older, do not isolate yourself. Surround yourself with helping hands: carers, nurses, people in your community.

2. **Stay active**
Keep doing things that matter to you. Whether it is work, hobbies, volunteering or learning something new, activity helps you stay connected and engaged.

3. **Get in shape**
Regular movement keeps the body strong and flexible. It can be as simple as walking, gardening, or stretching. As you age, do not stop moving. Even if you only move your little finger: move it.

4. **Take it slow**
Rushing makes it harder to notice the small things that give meaning. Moving at a gentler pace allows space for enjoyment and reflection.

5. **Eat in moderation**
The idea of eating until you are about 80 per cent full supports good health.

6. **Smile and acknowledge others**
Small gestures of kindness and connection, a smile, a greeting, a thank you, help build goodwill and a sense of belonging.

7. **Connect with nature**
Time in natural surroundings can lift mood, reduce stress and renew energy. This might be a walk in a park, time in a garden, or simply noticing the sky and trees.

8. **Give thanks**
Gratitude shifts attention to what is already good in your life.

A daily habit of noticing and appreciating can deepen your sense of meaning. Think about things you are grateful for. Some people make this into a daily meditation.

9. **Live in the moment**

Being present allows you to fully experience what is happening now, rather than being lost in regrets about the past or worries about the future. If you're feeling pain, pay attention to the pain. Feel its ebbing and flowing instead of blocking it out constantly.

10. **Follow your ikigai**

Spend time on the activities, roles and relationships that give you a reason to get up in the morning. Your ikigai may change over time, so keep exploring what brings you alive.

7

Blue Zones

B lue Zones are regions in the world where people live noticeably longer and healthier than the global average. The term was introduced by Dan Buettner, a National Geographic Fellow, who worked with researchers to identify and study these areas. The name originates from the blue circles the researchers drew on maps to mark the locations.

Five Blue Zones have been identified:

Okinawa, Japan – known for a plant-based diet, strong social connections, and a cultural emphasis on purpose, or ikigai.

Sardinia, Italy – particularly the mountain villages, where active daily routines, close family ties, and a Mediterranean diet are common.

Nicoya Peninsula, Costa Rica – noted for outdoor physical activity, a diet rich in beans and corn, and a strong sense of community.

Ikaria, Greece – famous for low rates of dementia and chronic illness, with a diet based on vegetables, legumes and olive oil, a relaxed daily rhythm, and a strong sense of community.

Loma Linda, California, USA – home to a large community of Seventh-day Adventists who follow a plant-based diet, avoid alcohol and smoking, and place importance on faith and social support.

Although each Blue Zone is unique in culture and geography, researchers found common lifestyle factors that seem to contribute to longevity and well-being. These include regular physical activity, a sense of purpose, strong community bonds, a plant-based diet, moderate calorie intake, and time spent with friends and family.

The Myth and the Reality

Okinawa, especially, is often presented as a timeless example of healthy living. Images of elderly women tending gardens, neighbours gathering to share food, and long lifespans are used to illustrate the benefits of ikigai and traditional ways of life. While these traditions still exist for some older Okinawans, they no longer represent the whole picture.

In recent decades, Okinawa has experienced rapid dietary and lifestyle changes. Western-style fast food has become common, and Okinawa now ranks among Japan's highest consumers of it. Younger generations are less likely to follow traditional diets, and rates of obesity and lifestyle-related diseases have risen. Car-based transport has replaced much of the natural daily movement that older generations maintained, and some of the tight-knit community structures have weakened.

This does not mean the lessons from Okinawa's past are invalid. The older generation, who grew up with traditional diets, active routines and strong community bonds, still show the benefits of those habits. However, it is important to recognise that the Okinawa of today is not the same as the Okinawa that inspired the idea of the Blue Zones.

8

Superagers

Some people in their seventies, eighties and beyond maintain the memory, attention and mental sharpness of those decades younger. Researchers call them *superagers*. They are not only mentally alert but often physically active, socially connected and full of curiosity.

Strong relationships and regular interaction with others have been linked to slower cognitive decline. Superagers often have active social lives, whether through friends, family, community groups or volunteering.

Researchers have found that superagers tend to have a thicker region of the brain's cortex in areas related to attention and memory. This may be partly genetic, but lifestyle also appears to make a difference. Mental challenge, physical activity and meaningful social connection all help preserve brain function.

Physical activity is another common factor. Superagers often stay active through walking, sports, dancing, swimming or other forms of movement they enjoy. Staying physically fit supports blood flow to the brain and keeps the body resilient.

Instead of settling into routines that require little effort, superagers engage in activities that demand focus, learning, and problem-solving. This might include studying a new language, playing a musical instrument, mastering a new skill, or engaging in challenging conversations and debates.

Superagers remind us that ageing does not have to mean decline only. By keeping the mind and body sharp and active, staying socially connected, and embracing challenges, it is possible to remain mentally sharp and engaged with life and community well into later years.

Good Ideas for Becoming a Superager

Stay socially connected

It is hard to overestimate the importance of social connections. Do not isolate yourself, even if you're in pain. Connect with providers of help and care if you're old or disabled. Keep in touch with friends and family, join groups, and meet new people. Regular conversation and connection help keep the mind sharp.

Move every day

Walk, swim, dance, garden or play a sport you enjoy. Regular movement supports both body and brain health. If you can only move your pinkie, move your pinkie.

Challenge your mind

Learn new skills, study a language, or take on mentally demanding hobbies. Avoid choosing the easiest path.

Mix up your routines

Try new routes, recipes, books or music. Variety keeps the brain active and flexible.

Eat for brain health

Include vegetables, fruit, whole grains, healthy fats and proteins. Limit processed foods and excess sugar.

Rest and recover

Give your body and brain the downtime they need with enough sleep and regular moments of calm.

Keep a sense of meaning

Find things that add meaning, be creative and/or part of something larger.

Eleven Years in Japan

I lived and worked in Japan for eleven years, from 1982 to 1993. This period coincided with the so-called economic bubble, a time when anything seemed possible. It was during those years that I first learned about ikigai.

The first time I heard the word was in calligraphy class with my teacher, whom I affectionately called Tomato-chan, due to her great fondness for tomatoes. I joined her class expecting merely to master brush strokes. Little did I know I was on the verge of discovering something far more important.

She would demonstrate, and I would imitate. Over months and eventually years, I observed her closely. She ground the ink with slow, deliberate care. She gripped the brush neither too firmly nor too loosely. With each stroke, she breathed life into the character. The emphasis lay not only on the final product, but on the act itself, the immersion in it.

One day after class, she remarked, "Suzanne-chan, *ikigai* is *kimochi*." *Kimochi* means feeling. Ikigai, she implied, arises from getting lost in what you are doing, guided by feeling.

That eventually became my approach to navigating the world: attentive, devoted, infused with kimochi.

Later, when I lost my ikigai, sprawled on the bed gazing at the unreachable yoga mat, it was the recollection of that feeling that summoned me back.

Ikigai transcends mere concept. It is a lived practice. Once experienced, its essence lingers indelibly.

The Flow State

The "flow state" is a term used to describe deep absorption in an activity. When you are in a state of flow, your attention is fully engaged, time seems to pass differently, and the activity feels both challenging and enjoyable. It is sometimes referred to as "being in the zone."

Psychologist Mihaly Csikszentmihalyi, who studied this state, found that it occurs when skills are well matched to the challenge at hand. If the task is too easy, boredom sets in. If it is too difficult, it leads to frustration and anxiety. Flow happens when focus is high and distractions fade into the background.

Many people experience a state of flow during activities such as painting, writing, music-making, or crafting. Others find it in sport, gardening, cooking, problem-solving, or work. The common element is that the activity is meaningful to the person, requires concentration, and offers a sense of progress or mastery.

Flow can be linked to ikigai because both involve a sense of engagement and satisfaction. Moments of flow contribute to a person's feeling that life has meaning. Even small periods of flow can create a sense of renewal and joy.

Creating opportunities for flow may involve choosing activities that are slightly beyond your comfort zone, removing distractions, and permitting yourself to be fully absorbed in the moment. It can be as simple as setting aside time for something you love and giving it your full attention.

While flow cannot be forced, it can be encouraged. By noticing the situations and activities where you naturally experience it, you can make space for more of these moments.

Flow does not need to be rare or reserved for significant achievements.

Small, regular experiences of flow can accumulate to create a greater sense of meaning. Cooking a meal, tending plants, repairing something, playing with a child, or losing yourself in a book can all bring this state of focused enjoyment. What matters is not the size or importance of the activity, but the quality of attention you give to it.

Flow is more likely when distractions are minimised. Turning off your phone, setting aside uninterrupted time, and creating a comfortable environment can help you focus more easily.

Choosing activities that match your skills and give you a clear goal also helps. The task should be engaging enough to hold your interest but not so difficult that it becomes stressful.

Finding flow is about more than enjoyment. It can strengthen resilience, reduce stress, and make ordinary routines more rewarding. Over time, these moments of engagement can contribute to your ikigai, helping you feel that your days are worthwhile.

By paying attention to where you already experience flow and making conscious choices to nurture it, you turn ordinary moments into opportunities for connection, creativity and a sense of fulfilment.

From Glow to Flow

Before entering a state of flow, there is a state that can be described as *glow*. Glow is the feeling of energy, enthusiasm and readiness that comes just before full immersion in an activity. It is a gentle build-up that warms you to the task and sets the stage for deeper focus.

Glow can feel like a spark of excitement, a sense of curiosity, or a rising eagerness to begin. You might feel it when you set up your paints before starting a painting, when you gather ingredients for a meal you are cooking, or when you open a book you have been wanting to read. It is the moment when you feel drawn in, but before time begins to disappear.

Recognising glow is essential because it is an opportunity to lean in and give yourself the conditions you need for flow.

Glow can be used as a guide. If a planned activity gives you no glow at all, it may not be the best choice for flow in that moment. Not every task will feel inspiring, but the activities that bring a little spark are often the ones most likely to lead to full engagement.

By noticing and nurturing glow, you prepare the ground for flow. Taking a few minutes to settle in, arrange your space, and connect with the intention behind what you are doing can turn an ordinary start into the gateway for a satisfying experience.

While flow can occur naturally, there are common barriers that make it more challenging to achieve. Some come from the environment, others from our own habits or mindset. Recognising these barriers is the first step toward removing them.

One obstacle is distraction. Constant interruptions from phones, email or other demands can keep attention from settling on one task. Incomplete focus makes it difficult to enter the state of deep engagement that flow requires.

Another barrier is a poor match between skill and challenge. If the activity is far too easy, you may feel bored. If it is far too hard, it can lead to frustration or anxiety. Flow needs the middle ground, where the task is engaging and just challenging enough to hold your attention.

A lack of meaning can also block the flow. If the activity feels meaningless or is done only out of obligation, it can be hard to give it full attention. Even necessary tasks can support flow if you connect them to a reason that matters to you.

Physical and mental fatigue can also play a role. Being stressed or unwell makes it harder to focus and to maintain the mental energy that flow requires. Rest and recovery are essential parts of creating the conditions for glow and flow.

Glow and flow happen when the mind and body feel safe enough to engage fully in the present. The opposite occurs when we feel threatened, unsafe or overwhelmed.

Survival states are freeze, flight, flop and fawn. They are natural, instinctive responses that help protect us in dangerous situations. However, when they become habitual, they can block the possibility of glow and flow.

Freeze: The body becomes tense and still. Attention narrows, and action feels impossible. This is like hitting pause in order to stay safe.

Flight: The urge is to escape. This may mean physically leaving a situation or mentally distracting yourself so you do not have to face it.

Flop: The body's energy drops suddenly. It goes limp or shuts down. There can be dissociation.

Fawn: The instinct is to please or appease others to avoid conflict or danger, even if it means ignoring your own needs.

These states are often triggered by trauma or repeated experiences of stress and pain. The nervous system learns to recognise certain situations as unsafe, even when the actual danger has passed. Over time, the body may slip into these responses automatically.

Somatic work provides gentle ways to shift out of these patterns. It focuses on the connection between mind and body, using awareness, breath, movement and sensation to restore a sense of safety. When the nervous system feels secure, the conditions for glow and flow return.

Understanding these survival states is not about judging yourself; it's about understanding yourself. They are signs that your body has been protecting you. The aim is to learn how to transition from these automatic responses into states of flow and glow.

12

Your Nervous System

Your nervous system connects your brain, spinal cord and nerves. It controls every function in your body, from movement and sensation to memory, emotion and decision-making. It also plays a central role in how you respond to stress and pain, as well as how you perceive safety. The nervous system has two main parts. The central nervous system includes the brain and spinal cord. It processes information and coordinates responses. The peripheral nervous system comprises all the nerves that branch out from the spinal cord to the rest of the body. It carries messages between the body and the brain.

The peripheral nervous system has a branch called the autonomic nervous system, which regulates functions you do not consciously control, such as breathing, heart rate, digestion and temperature. The autonomic nervous system has two main divisions: The sympathetic nervous system activates the body in response to stress. It increases heart rate, sends blood to the muscles, and releases energy so you can respond to a challenge or threat. This is sometimes referred to as the "fight or flight" system. The parasympathetic nervous system calms the body after stress. It slows the heart rate, supports digestion, and restores balance. This is sometimes referred to as the "rest and digest" system.

When you feel safe, these two systems work together. You can be alert and active when needed, and you can rest and digest when the challenge has passed. However, if you experience pain, trauma or prolonged stress, the nervous system can become dysregulated. It may stay in a state of high alert, or it may shut down to protect you. Over time, this can affect mood, energy, health and the ability to feel connected to yourself and others. Learning how your nervous system works is the first step in caring for it. With awareness, it is possible to bring it back into balance, allowing you to respond to life with greater flexibility and a deeper sense of safety. This, in turn, will return you to glow and flow.

13

Reset Your Nervous System

A well-regulated nervous system can move smoothly between states of activity and rest. You can respond to challenges with energy and focus, and then return to a calm, steady state once the challenge has passed.

When the nervous system becomes dysregulated, it may remain in a state of high alert, which can manifest as anxiety, restlessness, or irritability. It can also swing toward shutdown, which can feel like exhaustion, numbness or withdrawal. These patterns often develop after trauma, prolonged stress or repeated overwhelm.

Regulation means helping the nervous system return to a state of balance. This is not about forcing yourself to relax. It is about creating the right conditions for your body and mind to feel safe. Over time, this allows the nervous system to respond flexibly rather than react automatically.

Simple ways to support regulation are described in the next chapters. There are eleven practices. You can start with one and add a new one each week.

Consistency is important. Small, regular practices are more effective than occasional efforts. Over time, these habits can rebuild a sense of stability and make it easier to experience both glow and flow.

Regulating the nervous system is a gradual process. It is not about never feeling stress or pain again. It is about having the capacity to return to balance so you can live, work and connect with others from a place of steadiness and safety.

I have found that, when recovering from pain, trauma or stress, the following resets are extremely helpful.

14

Session 1: Moving the Eyes

This simple activity, developed by Stanley Rosenberg, can help calm your nervous system by stimulating the vagus nerve. It is often used as a gentle first step in somatic work when you are beginning to reconnect with a sense of safety in your body.

Here's how to do it:

Lie comfortably on your back or sit in a chair. Interlace your fingers and place your hands behind your head. Keep your elbows open to the sides.

Without moving your head, shift your gaze as far to one side as you can. Do not strain; move them to a comfortable limit.

Hold your gaze there for 30–60 seconds, or until you feel like yawning, swallowing, sighing, or coughing.

Bring your eyes back to the centre.

Repeat the same eye movement to the other side and hold.

Close your eyes and observe your body; feel the inside of it. This is called integration. It is as essential as the activity itself.

The movement of the eyes, while the head stays still, gently activates the part of the nervous system that helps the body relax. Some people feel the effect immediately, they begin to yawn, sigh, stretch their arms and chest. . . For others, it is more subtle. If you notice no change at first, that is fine; the activity is still beneficial.

You can use this activity as a brief break during the day or as a starting point for other somatic practices. The aim is to help the body register that it is safe enough to shift toward a state of rest and digest.

This activity only takes a couple of minutes.

You can expand it by letting your head rest on your shoulder and placing your hand on your head.

There are many demonstrations of Stanley Rosenberg's eye movement exercise on YouTube.

15

Session 2: Block Breathing

I f you have noticed some glimpses of relaxation, no matter how small, from last week's eye movements and started shifting from a freeze state toward more wellness, keep going. If not, be patient; it will come. Begin with the eye movements. Then move on to what you're going to learn next.

Block breathing is a simple way to calm the nervous system and bring focus to the present moment. It is sometimes called box breathing. It helps reduce stress and creates a sense of steadiness.

Here's how to do it:

Sit, lie down, or stand.
Breathe in through your nose for a slow count of four.
Hold your breath for a slow count of four.
Breathe out gently through your mouth for a slow count of four.
Hold your breath again for a slow count of four.
Repeat the cycle.

Keeping the counts even is important. The steady rhythm signals to the body that it is safe to relax. If four counts feels too long, you can start with three and gradually increase as it becomes easier.

You can do this as long as you like. I did it for twenty minutes just after my backache attack, because it was so soothing. I slowly reduced the time as I increased the somatic activities. It is up to you.

Block breathing can be used almost anywhere. With regular use, it can become a quick and reliable way to reset your nervous system.

You now have two activities to do a day:

1. Moving the eyes to the side while keeping the face still.
2. Block breathing 4/4/4/4

16

Session 3: Tapping and Mapping

I f you have already experienced glimpses of well-being and begun shifting from a freeze state toward greater wellness, continue with this activity. If you have not yet noticed such shifts, remain patient. They can take time to emerge.

This week's practice combines tapping with the eye movement and block breathing activities you have already learned.

Here's how it works:

Begin with the back of your hand. Lightly tap your skin with your fingertips while saying, out loud or silently: *This is me. This is my skin. This is my boundary.*

Some people notice sensation immediately. Others may feel numbness. If sensation is absent in the tapped area, gently scrape the skin with your nails while repeating: *This is me. This is my skin. This is my boundary.*

Tap and/or scrape the entire body this way. From time to time, look directly at the body part you are tapping or scraping. Over the week, you can gradually map the skin's full surface, noticing which areas feel sensitive and which seem numb.

In the following weeks, progress from tapping to gently squeezing the skin. Use a soft grip and continue repeating: *This is me. This is my skin. This is my boundary.*

After each session, wrap yourself in a blanket or a sheet and, with your eyes closed, feel what this does to your body.

The sequence of tapping or scraping, and squeezing, and finally wrapping yourself in a blanket offers a sense of safety. These steps help to address the numbness or disconnection often experienced in freeze states. Connecting with the skin, the body's primary boundary, supports a stronger sense of security. The combination of words and sensory input anchors this process, encouraging integration.

With regular practice, this activity helps lay the foundation for greater well-being, glow and flow.

Your daily routine now consists of:

1. Eye movements to the left and to the right
2. Block breathing 4/4/4/4
3. Tapping, scraping, and/or squeezing the skin
4. Wrapping yourself

17

Session 4: Hello Gravity

Paying attention to the pull of gravity on your body helps bring your focus away from your head and into your body. To be well, you need to be able to feel with your body.

Here is how it works:

Sit or lie down in a comfortable position. Close your eyes and let your breathing settle. Spend a few minutes doing the eye movements, block breathing, and tapping.

Next, notice how gravity is pulling on your body. Feel the weight in your head, shoulders, arms, hands, chest, belly, hips, upper legs, knees, lower legs, and feet.

Sense the weight and shape of your body. Notice how it presses into whatever is supporting it.

You can do this practice at any time and in any place, sitting at a desk, standing in a queue, or lying in bed.

There is a difference between knowing about gravity and actually feeling it. This shift from understanding to sensation takes practice for some. Time for integration, doing nothing with your eyes closed, observing the body, is just as important as the practice itself.

Research shows that grounding activities like this reduce anxiety and improve body awareness. Feeling gravity helps anchor you in the present moment, an important step in moving out of freeze states.

In trauma recovery, the term "container" refers to your ability to hold and manage emotions and sensations without becoming overwhelmed. Building a strong container happens gradually, through small and consistent steps.

Grounding in Gravity

Choose comfort first
Sit, stand, or lie in a position where your body feels supported.

Start with the other practices
Use eye movements, block breathing, or tapping to help you settle before focusing on gravity.

Scan from head to toe
Bring awareness to each part of your body and notice its weight.

Let yourself feel supported
Pay attention to the contact between your body and the surface beneath you.

Practice anywhere
Try this while sitting at a desk, standing in a queue, or resting in bed.

Keep it short and frequent
A few minutes repeated often works better than long, occasional sessions.

Allow time to integrate
After the practice, pause and notice how your body feels without rushing to the next activity.

If you have enough mobility, you can extend this practice to swaying in a standing position.

Bend your knees slightly.

Plant your feet at shoulder width on the ground and lightly sway like a tree in the wind in all directions.

Be aware of your *Ki,* the middle point of your body, an area deep in the body, just below the navel.

Close your eyes if you can and keep swaying lightly like a tree in the wind.

You now have the following activities in your daily routine:

1. Eye movements to the left and to the right
2. Block breathing 4/4/4/4
3. Tapping, scraping, and squeezing the skin
4. Feeling gravity while lying down, sitting or swaying while standing
5. Wrapping yourself
6. Recording glimmers of well-being

18

Recognising and Recording Glimmers

When living with pain or recovering from stress or trauma, it is easy to notice the moments when discomfort or tension increases. What often goes unnoticed are the moments when the body and mind feel lighter, calmer, or more at ease. These moments are called *glimmers*.

The previous four activities are so powerful that they alone can significantly increase your glimmers.

A glimmer is the opposite of a trigger. It is a signal from the nervous system that you are safe, even if only for a few seconds. You might feel a deeper breath, notice a softening in your muscles, or experience a sense of peace. It could be the warmth of sunlight on your face, the sound of a bird, a shared laugh, or a memory that makes you smile.

These glimmers are subtle, especially if pain or stress has been present for a long time. With practice, your attention shifts more easily toward these moments of well-being.

When you notice a glimmer, your nervous system gets a message that not all is threat or discomfort. This helps to interrupt the constant loop of pain signals and stress responses. By giving attention to glimmers, you train your brain to recognise safety and calm more often, which can gradually reduce the intensity and frequency of pain.

- Pay attention to changes in your breath, posture, or muscle tone
- Notice moments of pleasant sensation, however small
- Tune into sights, sounds, smells, or touches that feel soothing
- Observe when your mind feels clear or focused, even briefly

Record glimmers as they happen. Notice how pain or stress comes in waves. How it ebbs and flows.

Write down what you were doing, what you noticed in your body. Over time, you will build a personal map of the activities, environments, and people that help you feel better. The more you acknowledge and record these moments, the easier it becomes to find them again. This is not about ignoring pain or pretending it is not there. It is about gently balancing your awareness, so that your nervous system learns that safety and comfort are also part of your daily experience.

Noticing Glimmers

Start small
Look for just one or two glimmers each day. Over time, they will become easier to spot.

Use all your senses
Pay attention to sights, sounds, smells, tastes, and textures that feel pleasant.

Notice changes in your body
A softer jaw, looser shoulders, or a fuller breath can signal a glimmer.

Pause when you find one
Stay with the feeling for a few seconds to let your body register it.

Write it down or record it
Keep a notebook or voice recorder handy to capture glimmers in the moment.

Some people stick stars to their bathroom mirror.

Review your list
Looking back on your glimmers can help you see patterns and remind you of what works.

Share with someone
Discussing your glimmers with a friend or therapist can strengthen the sense of connection and safety they provide.

Your daily routine now contains:

1. Eye movements to the left and to the right
2. Block breathing 4/4/4/4
3. Tapping, scraping, and squeezing the skin
4. Wrapping yourself
5. Recognising glimmers of well-being

Example of Glimmer Record

29 November 2024

I was yawning in a lazy cat type of way all through the afternoon. It was a good feeling. Relaxed.

The block breathing is the most soothing for my pain situation. I spent a long time doing it this morning and experienced several moments of well-being during and after it.

Tapping the skin and acknowledging it as a boundary can be very powerful. I did it for a long time and identified several areas that are numb.

The wrapping in a blanket or sheet: I don't see the point, but I do it anyway.

All together, I walk a little better each day. This in itself is fantastic.

19

Session 5: Inner-Body Scan

This is the fifth session of your somatic practices. The previous four activities are so powerful that they alone can significantly increase your glimmers.

Have you noticed any glimmers of well-being? Have you been recording them?

Somatic practices are about reconnecting with your body after trauma, stress, or overwhelm, for example, when in pain.

This week's focus is the *inner-body scan*.

Begin with your regular practice. Then start the new activity by lightly tapping your hand. Close your eyes while keeping your awareness on that hand. If the sensation fades when your eyes are closed, open them again to bring it back. Tap once more, close your eyes, and sense the inner feeling of aliveness in the hand.

What do you notice? It might be warmth, tingling, throbbing, or a glow.

Stay with your attention on whatever you are feeling in the hand.

Then switch to the other hand and do the same. Feel the aliveness.

You can extend this to as many body parts as you wish. The more areas you explore, the more complete the scan will be. A simple way is to start at the feet and work gradually up to the head. You do not have to tap everywhere. As soon as you are able to direct your attention to a body part with your eyes closed, you can cease the tapping.

The inner-body scan directs attention inward to observe sensations. It is related to the traditional body scan meditation found in ancient Indian practices. In the West, it has been adapted in approaches such as mindfulness-based stress reduction.

From a polyvagal perspective, this practice encourages ventral vagal activation, which supports feelings of safety and connection. It helps widen your "window of tolerance", the range in which you can manage stress and emotions.

You now have the following activities in your daily routine:

1. Eye movements to the left and to the right
2. Block breathing 4/4/4/4
3. Tapping, scraping, and squeezing the skin
4. Feeling gravity while lying down, sitting or swaying while standing
5. Inner-body scanning
6. Wrapping yourself
7. Recording glimmers of well-being

You can spend as much or as little time on this sequence as you like. In case you need guidance, do the following:

Eye movements: 1 minute left, 1 minute right, 1 minute integration.

Block breathing: 10 rounds of in/hold/out/hold.

Tapping, scraping, squeezing: Do a body part per session, for example: head and face, arm and shoulder, upper body front, etc. 3 minutes.

Feeling gravity: lying down 1 minute, sitting, 1 minute, standing 1 minute.

Inner body scan: 5 minutes.

Wrapping yourself: 1 minute.

Total: 25 minutes

Don't forget to record your glimmers.

20

Session 6: Trembling and Shaking

I hope you have continued your practices. May your glimmers of well-being continue to grow.

Do not underestimate the power of the small activities you have been doing and the one you are going to do today.

Today's session's addition is *trembling and shaking*.

Here is how it works:

After your regular practices, lie down, close your eyes, and breathe steadily. Begin to tremble and shake your whole body. If that feels too much, start with your arms and hands, then gradually include other areas until your whole body is moving. Keep the movements small and light; do not progress them too violently.

Trembling and shaking help to release trapped survival energy, much like animals do after a threat has passed. This supports the resetting of the nervous system. It is built into our biology and plays an important role in restoring homeostasis, or balance, in the body.

When an animal senses danger, its autonomic nervous system activates the sympathetic branch. This prepares the body for fight or flight by increasing heart rate, speeding up breathing, and releasing adrenaline. Once the danger has passed, the animal will shake to discharge the leftover stress energy.

In humans, social conditioning often suppresses this instinct, leaving the body with unresolved tension that can contribute to anxiety, stress, or physical symptoms.

Trembling and shaking encourages this natural discharge to complete the stress cycle and restore nervous system regulation.

Your daily routine now looks like this

1. Eye movements to the left and to the right
2. Block breathing 4/4/4/4
3. Tapping, scraping, and squeezing the skin
4. Feeling gravity while lying down, sitting or swaying while standing
5. Inner-body scanning
6. Trembling and shaking
7. Wrapping yourself
8. Recording glimmers of well-being

Avoid thinking of these as obligations. Instead, look for ways to make them enjoyable. These practices are helping you move from freeze, toward glow, and ultimately into flow, as you reawaken and regulate your nervous system.

21

Session 7: Grounding and Centring

This week revolves the body's centre, located just below the belly button, deep within the belly toward the spine. This represents an area rather than a precise point, known as *hara* or *Ki* in martial arts traditions.

Perform this practice while standing with your feet positioned beneath your shoulders and slightly apart, knees relaxed rather than locked. If needed, use a walking frame for support. Direct your attention to the hara. Sense how gravity is pulling on your feet.

Shift your weight slightly forward, then back, left, right, noticing when you feel off-centre and when you feel centred.

Find your centre and sway gently like a tree in the wind, staying centred. It is a very small movement. Apply this to various body parts, shifting out of the centre and back. Remember to keep breathing.

Spend as long as feels comfortable with this swaying while feeling the hara.

This practice differs from the first swaying like a tree in the wind activity because you can use different body parts, for example, only your arm, or only your head.

Grounding and centring practices like these enhance stability, reduce anxiety, and foster a deeper bodily connection.

Your routine now includes:

1. Eye movements to the left and to the right
2. Block breathing 4/4/4/4
3. Tapping, scraping, and squeezing the skin
4. Feeling gravity while lying down, sitting or swaying while standing
5. Inner-body scanning
6. Trembling and shaking
7. Swaying and coming back to the centre
8. Wrapping yourself
9. Recording glimmers of well-being

22

Session 8: Sound Breathing

This chapter adds another breathing variation: sound breathing. You can do this in any comfortable position. Begin by focusing on your breath and making the exhalation longer than the inhalation.

Creating a gentle sound in your throat, such as *hhhhaaaa* or *sssssss*. This helps to slow and lengthen the exhalation, which, in turn, activates the parasympathetic response.

Sound breathing supports relaxation, helps prepare the body for sleep, counters insomnia, and promotes emotional balance and overall well-being. It also helps to ease physical tension.

Sound Breathing

Choose a comfortable position
Sit, lie down, or stand in a way that feels supported and relaxed.

Focus first
Take a moment to notice your breathing before you begin.

Lengthen the outbreath
Make the exhalation longer than the inhalation to calm your system.

Add a sound
Use a gentle sound like *hhhhaaaa* or *sssssss* to slow and smooth the
outbreath.

Release tension
As you exhale, soften the body.

Keep it flexible
Aim for ten in and out breaths, longer if possible.

Your routine now includes:

1. Eye movements
2. Block breathing
3. Tapping, scraping, and squeezing
4. Feeling gravity
5. Scanning the inner body
6. Trembling and shaking
7. Grounding and centring
8. Sound breathing to prolong the outbreath
9. Using the blanket for containment
10. Noticing glimmers of well-being

You can now begin to shorten those activities that feel most inte-
grated.. Around twenty minutes for all activities can serve as a mini-
mum, but there is no maximum.

23

Session 9: Pendulation and Titration

This chapter focuses on pendulation and titration.

Pendulation is designed to facilitate the nervous system's natural movement between states of activation, tension, or stress, and states of deactivation, calm, or safety, allowing for rest and digestion.

Titration means approaching difficult material in small, manageable doses to prevent overwhelm.

In somatic experiencing as we are practising here, these techniques allow the release of stored trauma energy gradually and safely. Pendulation creates a rhythm between distress and calm, while titration ensures that contact with challenging sensations or memories happens in a controlled, incremental way. Used together, they enable the processing of trauma and pain without triggering overload, allowing the nervous system to regulate and restore balance.

Here's how it works:

Lie down and breathe deeply. Slowly scan your inner body for areas that feel comfortable, beginning with your head and moving down through the neck, shoulders, arms, hands, chest, belly, hips, upper legs, knees, lower legs, and feet.

When you locate a comfortable area, rest your attention there and sense it fully. Then shift to an uncomfortable or painful area, staying only briefly before returning to the safe one.

This back-and-forth is called *pendulation*.

Repeat the process, gradually increasing the time you spend with the tense or painful area until it begins to feel more at ease. You can apply this to as many body parts as you wish.

You can also use pendulation and tritration with memories. This works as follows:

Recall a safe or pleasant memory and immerse yourself in its details. Then move to a mildly tense, unsafe, or uncomfortable memory, staying only momentarily before returning to the safe one. Repeat, slowly extending the time with the tense memory. With persistence, these memories often lose some of their charge and become easier to hold.

Finish by closing your eyes and noticing your body's overall state after the practice.

Your daily routine now contains:

1. Eye movements
2. Block breathing
3. Tapping, scraping, and squeezing
4. Feeling gravity
5. Scanning the inner body
6. Trembling and shaking
7. Grounding and centring
8. Sound breathing to prolong the outbreath
9. Pendulation and tritation

10. Using the blanket for containment
11. Noticing glimmers of well-being

24

Session 10, Spreading Your Toes

This chapter adds spreading your toes to your toolkit.

Lie down and breathe steadily. Focus on your feet and spread your toes apart, holding the position for a few seconds before relaxing. Repeat several times. Scrunch or curl your toes between spreads for balance.

If you cannot spread your toes at all, keep trying. Look at your feet. Try one foot at a time. Place your foot on your knee, so it's closer to your brain and try again.

This is a critical activity. The signal from your brain travels through the body from head to toe.

If you cannot spread your toes, after several weeks of trying, use toe spacers. Toe socks are good too. These simple tools help retrain the feet. Wear them while resting or walking around the house.

You can also use your fingers to spread your toes. This encourages the whole body to remain soft and flexible while you reach for your feet.

Spreading your toes helps restore toe alignment, which is often compromised by modern footwear. It strengthens the muscles of the feet, improves arch support, and enhances stability during walking or standing. This reduces the risk of falling.

In a somatic context, toe spreading increases body awareness, helps release tension, and reconnects you with the lower body. This supports better posture and more efficient movement. Overall, it is a simple yet powerful way to maintain mobility and well-being.

Your daily routine now looks like this:

1. Eye movements
2. Block breathing
3. Tapping, scraping, and squeezing
4. Feeling gravity
5. Scanning the inner body
6. Trembling and shaking
7. Grounding and centring
8. Sound breathing to prolong the outbreath
9. Pendulation and tritation
10. Spreading your toes
11. Using the blanket for containment
12. Noticing glimmers of well-being

25

Session 11: Dancing with the Arms

This final practice brings relaxation and an element of play to your sequence. Lie down in a comfortable position. Close your eyes and breathe steadily.

Begin to let your arms move gently through space, as if they were seaweed swaying in water. Allow the movements to be slow and unhurried, with no fixed pattern. The water can shift direction, grow stronger or softer — follow these imagined changes with your arms. Let your hands lead the way, and bring your full attention to their movement. Allow your arms to drift, pause, and change direction as they wish. Bring enjoyment to the movement.

This gentle, playful movement encourages relaxation, enhances body awareness, and invites a sense of freedom into your practice.

You now have a rich set of daily practices:

1. Eye movements
2. Block breathing
3. Tapping, scraping, and squeezing the skin
4. Feeling gravity and the body's weight
5. The body scan

6. Trembling and shaking
7. Sound breathing
8. Pendulation and titration
9. Spreading the toes
10. Dancing with the arms
11. Wrapping yourself in a blanket
12. Recording glimmers of well-being

Together, these practices help you move from freeze to glow and flow. They release stored tension, expand your capacity to feel safe, and strengthen your connection with your body. You can do the entire sequence or select practices as needed, knowing that each contributes to nervous system regulation and well-being. Do them daily until you naturally feel inclined to move toward more demanding activities.

In my case, it took about three months to establish a more demanding routine.

If you like this somatic work as much as I do, a part 2 to this book is in the making.

26

The Notion of Meaning

So far, we have explored the meaning of ikigai, from its Japanese roots in daily routines and relationships to its Western view as a pathway to purpose and flow. We have examined ten good ideas, along with a few additional ones, for rebuilding a meaningful life. We have also examined the myths and realities of Blue Zones and superagers and reflected on the lessons I learned during my eleven years in Japan. Along the way, we have considered the connection between ikigai and the states of glow and flow.

If you are living with burnout, pain, trauma, or stress, the idea of meaning may feel distant or out of reach. The somatic practices in this book are designed to create a sense of safety, opening the way to greater well-being. By tuning in to your nervous system, you create the conditions where meaning can take root, glow can grow, and flow can emerge.

In the days, weeks, or months ahead, depending on the speed with which you are reading this book, we will continue to explore the idea of meaning while you maintain your somatic practices.

Once you have become familiar with the somatic practices, they can be adapted to many different situations. During my recovery from the back pain episode described earlier in the book, I gradually wove them into my bath time routine. A short daily ritual, such as feeling the warmth of the water while practising skin tapping or block breathing, can help reinforce the body–mind connection. Warm water itself supports relaxation by dilating blood vessels, improving circulation, and lowering muscle tension, which can make somatic practices more effective.

When you feel ready, start incorporating regular physical activities that align with your interests and energy levels. In my own routine, I now use a rebounder (a small trampoline) and a Pilates reformer to help maintain my mobility. This is guided by the principle: "if you do not use it, you lose it." Rebounding offers gentle yet effective cardiovascular exercise while reducing joint strain. It can also improve lymphatic circulation, balance, and core strength. The Pilates reformer strengthens muscles, improves posture, and builds flexibility, all of which can counteract the effects of pain, stress, trauma or fatigue from past injuries. However, everyone has their own preferences, and I am not at all pushing Pilates or rebounding. Swimming or walking can be great too. It is entirely up to you. If you have a disability, move what you can move.

A central part of moving toward flow and rediscovering your ikigai, so you once again know what is worth getting up for in the morning, is nurturing both movement and, above all, social connection. Movement stimulates the release of endorphins and other neurotransmitters, such as dopamine and serotonin, which enhance mood and resilience. Social connection, meanwhile, plays an equally vital role in regulating the nervous system. Safe, enjoyable relationships activate the ventral vagal branch of the parasympathetic system, signalling to the body that it is safe, which promotes repair and restoration.

This deserves a prominent place on your priority list. In fact, large-scale studies such as the Harvard Study of Adult Development, the longest-running study of human happiness, have found that the quality of our relationships is the most critical factor for health and longevity. It ranks higher than diet, exercise, or genetics. Data from the Blue Zones also show that strong social networks, community engagement, and a sense of belonging are consistent traits among the world's longest-lived and healthiest populations.

Adding social elements to your movement can amplify the benefits. Walking with a friend, joining an exercise class, or participating in a shared hobby group combines physical activity with connection, creating a feedback loop that supports both mental and physical well-being. Social interaction is not just "nice to have" but a core biological need that influences everything from immune function to pain perception. Movement and connection form the foundation for sustained glow and flow. They help you find daily enjoyment and continue living a life worth living.

27

Joy

Do you know what brings you joy? For many, the memory of it has faded. It is worth asking yourself: *What truly brings me enjoyment?*

Tasks that are too easy feel dull. Those that match your skills—demanding but achievable—bring flow. Activities that are far beyond your abilities cause anxiety. The sweet spot is engaging without being overwhelming.

Set aside days or even weeks to think about this question. Be honest and write down what you find.

Self-Determination Theory emphasises the significance of intrinsic motivation—doing something for its own sake, for the sheer pleasure of it. Such activities often sustain interest far more than those done for money or praise.

Research on flow shows that when challenge and skill align, self-consciousness diminishes and motivation increases. Brain studies confirm that flow activates the brain's reward centres and quiets overthinking.

Memories of joy can fade if not revisited. Reflection reawakens them. Writing about joyful moments and trying new activities can strengthen this effect.

Taking the time to identify what brings you enjoyment is more than a pleasant exercise. It is a way to improve your mental health, motivation, and overall sense of meaning.

28

Intention

Before anything else, there is intention.
Intention is a quiet inner movement, a leaning toward something we value or desire. It is not the same as a goal or a plan. It doesn't ask for immediate action. It appears as a wish, a readiness, or a longing. It may lead to action, or it may simply need to be felt.

Intention changes the brain even before we take a single step. Forming an intention activates new possibilities in the nervous system, prepares the body for action and opens the way for change.

In healing from stress, illness, pain, or trauma, intention can be the first step. You may not yet be ready to speak, move, or feel difficult emotions, but you can form an inner statement such as "I want..." or "I feel like. . . "

We often rush from intention into action. Yet there is value in the space between. Holding intention without acting allows the nervous system to settle. It is like planting a seed; it needs time to take root before it can grow.

Try setting an intention for rediscovering your *ikigai*, your sense of purpose and joy. Keep it simple and personal. Let it rest. Let it breathe. Notice where you feel it, in your chest, your belly, or your hands.

There is no need to act. Just sit with it. Over time, it may guide you. You may notice small shifts in your choices, dreams, breathing, or movement. For now, let it exist. If you wish, write it down. But most importantly, let it live within you.

Neurologically, intention is a measurable brain process that prepares the body for voluntary action. It has clear neural signatures. Readiness potential begins more than half a second before we are consciously aware of our decision to move. This activity starts in the supplementary motor area and premotor cortex, which plan movement before it occurs, and is followed by the primary motor cortex to execute the action.

Intention primes neural circuits, increases readiness, and creates a foundation for action, even if no action follows. Repeated over time, forming an intention can create neuroplastic changes, strengthening the brain pathways it engages. Even imagining a movement can activate the same brain regions as performing it.

So, for now, dwell only on your intention, not on the action that may come after.

29

Ikigai-kan

What elements in your life, no matter how small, bring you a sense of well-being? What motivates you to get up in the morning? What forms of *ikigai-kan,* the feeling that life is worth living, already exist in your daily life? Consider making a list.

Your *ikigai-kan* might come from a child or grandchild, or from watching trees sway in the breeze. It could be savouring Spanish food, playing a game, painting, or arranging flowers. Perhaps it comes from listening to your favourite music, admiring sculptures, spending time with your daughter, or working at your computer. Watching YouTube videos, brewing beer, building houses, practising yoga, growing roses, or simply lying in bed could all evoke it. So could cooking, writing, styling hair, dancing ballet, working as a doctor, or spending time in a shed full of tools. Maybe it comes from indigo fabrics, playing the piano, cleaning, drawing with ink, sweeping, studying at university, driving, skipping rope, caring for a pet, nursing others, working as a plumber, ice skating, walking a tightrope, making ceramics, sitting in the sun, or enjoying Korean boy bands. . .

The point is that almost anything can hold the potential to spark your *ikigai-kan.*

Challenge yourself to find one hundred things that give your life meaning right now. If this feels difficult, pause and return to the somatic practices to help cultivate more glimmers of well-being. Avoid rushing into action if it still feels too demanding.

Move back and forth between your somatic practices and add to your *ikigai-kan* list, the things that make it worthwhile to get up in the morning.

30

Objectives

Once your social connections have strengthened and your nervous system has settled into a state of calm, accompanied by a growing sense of well-being, you are ready to move to the next phase of discovering your ikigai: identifying your objectives.

Objectives are goals such as moving house or obtaining a degree. Objectives differ from intentions. Intentions are broad, adaptable, and open-ended. They form the foundation, like seeds planted. Objectives are more defined and structured — the young plants emerging from those seeds, shaped by clarity and purpose.

Take your time with this stage. Ask yourself: What are my objectives? Make a list.

Once you have your list, sort your objectives into three categories:

Objectives that are vague and lack a clear process.

Objectives that are clearly defined and focus strongly on the process.

Objectives that you feel obsessed with, but where the process is missing or unclear.

Look at the vague objectives. Notice how they feel confusing or undefined. Try to name that confusion more precisely. Can you find clearer words to describe what you want? If you can bring these objectives into focus, do so. If not, set them aside for now.

Next, examine the obsessive objectives. These are the ones you may fixate on, but without knowing how to move toward them. Put effort into identifying the process that might lead you there. If a workable process does not emerge, let the objective rest for the time being.

Lastly, focus on the process-driven objectives — the ones that are clearly defined and grounded in actionable steps. This is where flow is most likely to arise. Glow and flow thrive when we have well-articulated goals that centre on process, not just the outcome.

Objectives built around a strong process bring many benefits:

1. They improve attention and concentration.
2. They support memory and learning.
3. They reduce the chance of errors.
4. They promote calmness and a sense of mastery.
5. They increase awareness of others.
6. They spark creativity.

Choose one or two of these objectives and begin working with them. If you start to feel overwhelmed, pause. Return to somatic practice. Then begin again when you are ready.

31

Glow and Flow Revisited

G low is an intermediate state of well-being that appears as the nervous system begins to move out of shutdown responses, such as freeze or flop, and shifts toward regulation and vitality. You may notice a gentle easing of muscular tension, slower and deeper breathing, or a sense of presence replacing numbness or dissociation. Glow does not yet fully capture the essence of flow, but it lays the essential groundwork. It reflects the reactivation of the ventral vagal state, the branch of the parasympathetic nervous system that supports social engagement, trust, and relational safety. Glow is not produced by effort but by repeated, gentle resets.

Glow must come before flow. It creates the physiological and emotional safety needed for meaningful engagement. Without glow, the nervous system may remain hypervigilant and unable to relax enough to take on purposeful or challenging activities. Trying to pursue ikigai or enter flow from a state of dysregulation often results in overwhelm. Glow acts as a bridge, widening the window of tolerance — the nervous system's capacity to manage stress — so that challenges feel stimulating rather than threatening. When glow becomes stable, it opens the way to flow.

Flow is a state of complete immersion in an activity, marked by focused attention, intrinsic motivation, and a sense of ease. In flow, the mind is fully absorbed in the present moment, undistracted by past concerns or future anxieties. Time may seem to slow or disappear. There is a feeling of agency and control, supported by preparation and clarity about the task at hand. Effort feels smooth and efficient, and actions unfold naturally. Often, the sense of self fades; it can feel less like you are doing the task and more like the task is moving through you.

If the mind is caught in past events or future worries, flow has not yet been reached, but glow may be present. Flow depends on the calm alertness that glow makes possible. It cannot be forced but arises when body and mind are synchronised — rooted in safety, supported by clarity, and attuned to the present.

32

Health

Your health provides a crucial foundation for rediscovering and sustaining your ikigai. When the body is well-nourished and cared for, the mind becomes clearer, energy more stable, and a deeper connection to purpose more accessible.

Begin with your diet. Prioritise whole, unprocessed foods over packaged or heavily refined products. Prepare meals from fresh ingredients. Cooking, baking, gardening, or foraging can strengthen your relationship with nourishment. If these options are not suitable for you, consider finding someone who can prepare nutritious food and pay for the service if necessary. Choose organic produce where possible. It tastes so much better. If meal preparation is challenging, ask for help from friends, family, neighbours, or community services. Proper nourishment is not a luxury — it is essential.

Reduce added sugars. When sweetness is desired, use natural alternatives such as honey, maple syrup, or (dried) fruits like figs and dates. Consider the Japanese principle of *harahachibu* — eating until you are about 80 per cent full.

Avoid tobacco and alcohol, as both disturb nervous system balance and undermine physical and emotional well-being.

Include regular movement in your daily life. This need not be intense exercise. Walking, stretching, gardening, swimming, dancing, or doing yoga all help maintain flexibility, mobility, and energy flow.

Movement supports mood, regulates hormones, and improves cardiovascular and cognitive health.

Approach these habits with enjoyment and connection. Share meals with others. Cook together. Move together. Health is not only a personal responsibility but also a relational and cultural practice. From a place of growing vitality and connection, your ikigai can take deeper root.

33

Growth

I rediscovered my ikigai after the severe episode of back pain described earlier in this book. My recovery began with somatic practices. Over time, I began to notice subtle signs of well-being. From there, I incorporated regular exercise into my routine and modified my diet, eliminating added sugar and processed foods. I began buying organic vegetables and fruit. I reflected on my intentions.

As I regained stability, I expanded my social life, sharing coffee and conversation with both old and new friends. I wrote down my objectives and mapped out the steps I needed to pursue them.

Writing this book became one of those objectives, and for a time, it was my ikigai. I kept enjoyment at the centre. What began as a backache evolved over nine months and continues to grow. While I still live with chronic back pain, I now experience flow daily.

Personal growth is valuable at any age and regardless of ability.

If you are feeling stuck, stressed, overwhelmed, distressed, or in persistent pain, seek support. You do not have to do this alone.

Throughout my life, ikigai and the flow state that often accompany it have helped me find fulfilment. I have followed what I love, often blurring the line between work and passion. I have travelled extensively, run three businesses, and recently completed a PhD. At 69, I remain active in my community, contributing through small acts of service. For example, I manage an online bulletin board that keeps locals informed about nearby events, sports and activities. I can do this while lying down if needed.

For the most part, life is fulfilling. And transformation, I have found, often begins with the smallest of steps, like moving your eyes.

34

Pain and Suffering

Meta-cognition, the capacity to reflect on one's own thinking, enables us to evaluate our plans and actions, develop strategies, and adapt behaviours. It enables learning, problem-solving, and decision-making.

Yet meta-cognition also marks the point at which pain is transformed into suffering. Unlike animals, who have a direct and immediate response to pain, humans can imagine alternatives — what might have been, what could happen, or what should be. . .

This distinction is echoed in the biblical story of the Garden of Eden. Before eating from the Tree of Knowledge, Adam and Eve lived in a state akin to that of animals — free of meta-cognition. After gaining meta-cognition, they became aware of themselves and others as separate beings, of unrealised possibilities, and with that awareness came shame, loss, and suffering.

Pain is the raw sensation, whether physical or emotional — the throb of a headache, the ache of grief. Suffering emerges when thoughts build a story around that pain: *This isn't fair, I can't function like this, I shouldn't feel this way after all I've done*. Such interpretations intensify the original discomfort.

Mental resistance heightens suffering, whereas acceptance reduces it. Mindfulness practices demonstrate this: By observing pain with curiosity and without judgment, we can separate the sensation from the narrative.

Recognising that suffering has meta-cognitive origins opens the way to relief. Observing thoughts without becoming entangled in them reduces the emotional load that pain carries. By noticing and reshaping unhelpful mental narratives, suffering can become more manageable — even meaningful, as in Japanese *gaman suru*.

Overanalysing can breed doubt or detachment, prompting questions like *Does this really matter?* or *Am I doing it right?* While such questions can be useful, they may also disrupt a sense of meaning if pursued excessively. Used with discernment, meta-cognition transforms obstacles into insight, strengthening resilience and clarity.

Hence, meta-cognition is double-edged. It elevates life from mere endurance to being enriched with direction, purpose, and ikigai-kan — the felt sense of meaning.

The Meaning of it All

I often hear the question: Does there have to be a meaning to life in general to live a meaningful personal life? I'll tell you the truth: I have no clue. I am fine living with "I don't know."

Or, if I really have to say something about the meaning of life, I go with Brian Cox, who says: "Life, just like the stars, the planets and the galaxies, is just a temporary structure on the long road from order to disorder. But that doesn't make us insignificant, because we are the Cosmos made conscious. Life is the means by which the universe understands itself. And for me, our true significance lies in our ability to understand and explore this beautiful universe."

And: "We are the cosmos made conscious, and life is the means by which the universe understands itself".

And: "The ingredients in our bodies were assembled in the hearts of long-dead stars over billions of years. These ingredients have spontaneously assembled into temporary structures that can think, feel, and explore."

Remember: Finding your ikigai is not about the meaning of life, but about finding meaning in *your* life.

Staying With It

You have reached the end of this book. There are no assessments to complete, no evaluations to pass, and no expectation of dramatic transformation.

Some ideas may have resonated with you, while others might have felt distant. This is natural. The path described here is not a technique to master, but a series of invitations, suggestions for exploration rather than prescriptions.

Take time to return to what moved you. Revisit what brought comfort or stability. This process does not end here. It unfolds over time, waiting patiently for your return. There may be periods when you forget, or when freeze returns. There is no rush, no timeline, no pressure. Begin again as often as needed.

Discovering your ikigai and entering a state of glow or flow does not guarantee permanence. Your emotional or physical state can shift, and with it, the sense of meaning.

I have experienced this myself when a once-vibrant connection to purpose and engagement diminished under the weight of stress and pain. These moments remind us that ikigai, like the nervous system it works alongside, needs ongoing care to stay alive.

Loss of ikigai often comes from imbalance, as I found in my own back pain story. Overload or underload, unrelenting demands, emotional strain, dissociation, or physical neglect can disrupt the delicate balance between body, mind, and environment.

In Japan, ikigai is nourished by the quiet constancy of routines and relationships; however, modern pressures can erode these, leading to disconnection.

In the Western view, ikigai arises from the meeting point of passion, skill, and need. When one of these falters — for example, through burnout, the whole structure weakens. Trauma, pain, chronic stress, or isolation can push us back into freeze or flop states, dimming glow and muting the ikigai-kan that makes mornings worth rising for.

Yet loss is not final. Each time I have drifted from my ikigai, I have returned by re-engaging with somatic experiencing. It helped to reset my nervous system, release tension, and reopen pathways to meaning.

In moments of disconnection, start small. Allow glimmers of well-being to reappear, and from them rebuild the conditions in which ikigai can grow again.

In the end, losing your ikigai shows its living, evolving nature.

And for those who want more somatic experiencing: Book 2 of Find Your Ikigai is in the making.

Accessibility Modifications for Somatic Exercises

The somatic practices described in this book are intended to be gentle and adaptable. Many people live with physical limitations, illness, or pain, and these activities must remain accessible to all. What follows are suggestions for adapting each practice. These are not medical recommendations; if you are uncertain, consult a healthcare professional before starting.

Week 1: Moving the Eyes

If lying on the floor is uncomfortable, sit in a supportive chair with your back and head well supported. You may also lie in bed with pillows behind your head and arms. If raising the arms behind the head is not possible, rest your hands on your lap or by your sides and simply move the eyes left and right without the hand position.

Week 2: Block Breathing

If sitting upright is difficult, practise block breathing while lying on your back with a pillow under your knees. If you cannot maintain an equal four-count rhythm, reduce to counts of two or three. If holding the breath is uncomfortable, omit the hold and instead focus on gentle inhalation and exhalation.

Week 3: Tapping and Mapping

If you have limited mobility, concentrate on accessible areas such as the arms, hands, or face. A soft cloth, sponge, or feather can be used instead of fingers. If the hands are weak or painful, ask a carer or friend to assist. For those with sensitivity issues, tapping can be replaced by resting the hand lightly on the skin and repeating the words silently.

Week 4: Hello Gravity

If standing is not safe, remain seated or lie down. Place cushions behind your back or under your legs so you feel supported. To adapt the swaying movement, imagine the sensation of swaying without moving the body. Even visualising gravity and the body's weight can promote a grounding effect.

Week 5: Inner-Body Scan

If tapping to bring sensation is too tiring, focus on a single body part such as the hands, feet, or face. The scan can be guided by imagination if the physical sensation is faint. For those with limited concentration, keep the scan very brief, returning to one or two familiar body areas.

Week 6: Trembling and Shaking

If lying down and shaking the whole body is not possible, choose a smaller movement such as trembling the hands, feet, or head. Even a light vibration in the tongue or lips can serve the same purpose. Some people find that imagining the body shaking provides relief when physical movement is limited.

Week 7: Grounding and Centring

If standing is not safe, this practice can be done in a seated position with feet flat on the floor. A chair with armrests provides stability. Small shifts forward, backward, and side to side can be visualised if actual movement is not possible. Placing a hand gently on the lower belly can help focus awareness on the hara.

Week 8: Sound Breathing

If producing a strong sound is difficult, exhale softly with a whisper or hum. Those with respiratory conditions can shorten the length of the exhalation and rest between rounds. Sound can also be imagined silently if vocalisation is not possible.

Week 9: Pendulation and Titration

If scanning the whole body is overwhelming, choose only two areas to move attention between, such as the hands and feet. For memory-based pendulation, use very mild and safe memories paired with a comforting image. If revisiting discomfort is too much, remain with the safe memory only.

Week 10: Spreading the Toes

If you cannot spread your toes actively, use your fingers to separate them. Toe spacers or toe socks can provide support without strain. If reaching the feet is difficult, ask a helper to assist or simply imagine the movement. Even visual attention to the feet can begin to create a brain–body connection.

Week 11: Dancing with the Arms

If lying down is not comfortable, this activity can be done seated or standing. If the shoulders are stiff, move only the hands or fingers in gentle swaying motions. If physical movement is very limited, imagine the arms as seaweed moving in water and follow the sensation in the mind.

Theoretical Foundations

This appendix looks more deeply at the principal theoretical frameworks that underpin this book: Polyvagal Theory, Somatic Experiencing, and Flow Theory. Together, they provide the scientific and psychological foundation for its approach to well-being, nervous system regulation, and the cultivation of ikigai. The sections below aim to give a clear and accessible overview, alongside suggestions for further reading.

Polyvagal Theory

Developed by Stephen Porges in the 1990s, Polyvagal Theory explains how the autonomic nervous system shapes social behaviour, emotional regulation, and physiological states through the vagus nerve. It describes a tiered system of responses to environmental cues and offers a framework for understanding how chronic stress or trauma can disrupt the nervous system, leading to states such as freeze or flop, and how somatic practices can restore balance.

The theory identifies three main states. The ventral vagal state, linked to social engagement, is activated in perceived safety. It supports social connection, emotional regulation, and bodily calm, often described as "rest and digest". Signs include a steady heart rate, relaxed breathing, open facial expressions, and a warm tone of voice. In relation to ikigai, this state fosters meaningful interaction and appreciation of daily pleasures. Practices such as sound breathing encourage it.

The sympathetic state mobilises the body when safety is uncertain, preparing for fight or flight. It is marked by increased heart rate, rapid breathing, heightened vigilance, and muscle tension. Prolonged sympathetic activation can lead to anxiety, restlessness, or exhaustion. In the context of ikigai, extended periods in this state can make it difficult to access the calm, present focus that supports ikigai-kan. Somatic practices help regulate this state.

The *dorsal vagal state* is the body's final response to overwhelming threat, bringing either freeze (stillness with heightened alertness) or flop (collapse, detachment, or shutdown). Signs include slowed heart rate, shallow breathing, emotional numbness, and dissociation. Somatic exercises such as trembling and shaking can help release trapped survival energy and restore adaptability.

Underlying these states is *neuroception*, the body's unconscious detection of safety or danger. Warm vocal tones or eye contact can stimulate the ventral vagus, while cues of threat shift the system toward sympathetic or dorsal states. Polyvagal Theory is widely applied in trauma therapy, education, and leadership, emphasising the importance of safety as the basis for engagement.

In this book, Polyvagal Theory clarifies freeze and flop states and informs practices such as tapping and grounding to restore ventral vagal tone. It also underscores the role of safe social connection, aligning with the Japanese emphasis on community as a pillar of ikigai.

Further reading: Stephen W. Porges, *The Polyvagal Theory: Neurophysiological Foundations of Emotions, Attachment, Communication, and Self-Regulation* (2011); Deb Dana, *The Polyvagal Theory in Therapy: Engaging the Rhythm of Regulation* (2018).

Deb Dana:
   The Polyvagal Theory in Therapy & Clinical Applications...
   Polyvagal Exercises for Safety and Connection; Polyvagal Flip Chart

Anchored: How to Befriend Your Nervous System
Polyvagal Card Deck: 58 Practices for Calm and Change
Polyvagal Practices: Anchoring the Self in Safety
Polyvagal Prompts: Finding Connection and Joy through Guided
Explorations; The Nervous System Workbook
Glimmers Journal: Reflect on the Small Moments

Somatic Experiencing

Created by Peter A. Levine, Somatic Experiencing is a body-based method for resolving trauma and chronic stress by focusing on physical sensations rather than retelling events. It sees trauma as incomplete physiological responses to threat, and aims to discharge trapped energy to restore balance in the nervous system. Levine emphasises that trauma arises not only from the event itself but from the body's inability to complete its natural survival responses. When fight, flight, or freeze is interrupted, the energy mobilised for action remains stuck, creating symptoms such as chronic pain, numbness, or anxiety.

Somatic Experiencing works with responses such as *freeze* (immobile alertness) and *flop* (deeper collapse and detachment), using tools like *titration* (addressing trauma in small doses to avoid overwhelm) and *pendulation* (moving attention between distressing and safe sensations). For example, shifting between tense and relaxed body areas in an inner-body scan can help integrate stored survival energy. Subtle movements or visualisations can complete interrupted defensive actions, restoring a sense of agency and safety.

The method strengthens *interoception* (awareness of internal sensations) and *proprioception* (awareness of body position), helping people reconnect with their bodies. Observing sensations such as warmth or tingling, and allowing spontaneous movements such as trembling, can release held energy and ease symptoms such as hyper-vigilance or pain.

In this book, Somatic Experiencing principles are adapted into accessible practices such as trembling, pendulation, and inner-body scanning to help readers move out of freeze or flop states and build resilience. The emphasis on completing survival responses aligns with ikigai by freeing energy for purpose and flow. The program's slow pace and focus on integration reflect Somatic Experiencing's priority of preventing overwhelm.

Further reading: Peter A. Levine, *Waking the Tiger: Healing Trauma* (1997); Peter A. Levine, *In an Unspoken Voice: How the Body Releases Trauma and Restores Goodness* (2010).

Flow Theory

Psychologist Mihaly Csikszentmihalyi introduced Flow Theory in the 1970s to describe a state of complete absorption in an activity, marked by deep focus, effortlessness, and intrinsic motivation. In flow, self-awareness recedes, time seems to disappear, and action feels seamless.

In this book, flow is linked to ikigai: purpose creates the condi-tions for flow, and flow in turn deepens the experience of ikigai. Flow is characterised by full immersion, a balance between challenge and skill, loss of self-consciousness, timelessness, and intrinsic reward. It arises when tasks are clear, challenging without overwhelming, pro-vide immediate feedback, and are undertaken with autonomy in an environment that supports focus.

Flow applies across contexts. In work, aligning tasks with ikigai can boost productivity and satisfaction. In art, it can dissolve time and connect the creator with inner passion. In sport, it underlies peak performance. In daily life, it can emerge in simple acts like gardening when approached with presence and engagement.

Flow's mechanisms involve neurochemicals such as dopamine for focus and endorphins for pleasure, as well as temporary downregulation of the prefrontal cortex, reducing self-consciousness and enabling intuitive action. Writers such as Steven Kotler, Brendon Burchard, and Cal Newport describe how environmental design, deep work habits, and energy management can foster flow. Somatic practices in this book, such as block breathing and inner-body scans, prepare the nervous system for flow by reducing stress and sharpening attention.

Further reading: Mihaly Csikszentmihalyi, *Flow: The Psychology of Optimal Experience* (1990); Steven Kotler, *The Art of Impossible: A Peak Performance Primer* (2021); Cal Newport, *Deep Work: Rules for Focused Success in a Distracted World* (2016).

Blue Zones

"Blue Zones" are geographical regions with unusually high concentrations of long-lived individuals, many of whom reach 90 or 100 years in good health. The concept was developed by demographer Michel Poulain and physician Gianni Pes, who mapped areas of exceptional longevity in Sardinia, using blue ink to mark them on demographic charts. The idea was later expanded and popularised by Dan Buettner in collaboration with National Geographic and the National Institute on Aging, identifying five regions: Okinawa (Japan), Sardinia (Italy), Nicoya (Costa Rica), Ikaria (Greece), and Loma Linda (California, USA).

Gianni Pes and Michel Poulain, *'Blue Zones: Areas of Exceptional Longevity Around the World'* (2004), which first introduced the terminology in a demographic context and focused on Sardinia.

Makoto Suzuki, Nobuyoshi Willcox and Craig Willcox, *The Okinawa Program: How the World's Longest-Lived People Achieve Everlasting Health—And How You Can Too* (Clarkson Potter, 2001), which documented dietary and lifestyle patterns of Okinawan centenarians.

Dan Buettner, *The Blue Zones: Lessons for Living Longer from the People Who've Lived the Longest* (National Geographic, 2008; revised editions 2012, 2015), synthesised findings across all identified regions and brought the concept into public health and policy discourse.

Dan Buettner, *The Blue Zones Solution: Eating and Living Like the World's Healthiest People* (National Geographic, 2015), applied the findings to lifestyle and nutrition practices for wider populations.

Superagers

Superagers are people, aged 80 or older, who display cognitive performance, especially in memory, that parallels that of individuals decades younger. They defy the usual narrative that cognitive decline is an inevitable consequence of ageing.

Neurological investigations reveal that Superagers:

1. Exhibit minimal cortical thinning, maintaining brain structure in key regions such as the anterior cingulate cortex.
2. Have increased density of von Economo neurons, which are implicated in social–emotional processing.
3. Display healthier entorhinal neurons in the hippocampus (key for memory) and clearer white matter microstructure, indicating resilience against age-related decline.
4. Resist or remain resilient to neuropathologies such as amyloid plaques and tau tangles, hallmarks of Alzheimer's disease.
5. Often show fewer activated microglia in the brain, potentially indicating a distinct immune environment
6. Demonstrate excellent performance in memory tests, for example, recalling at least 9 out of 15 words on delayed recall, equating them cognitively with individuals aged 50–60.

Superagers tend to be socially engaged, autonomous, and cognitively active, traits that may support cognitive resilience, even when lifestyle habits otherwise vary.

Research into Superagers originates from longitudinal studies, such as the one at Northwestern University, that have monitored well-characterised individuals and conducted brain donation studies to elucidate their neurobiological underpinnings.

In sum, Superagers exemplify exceptional cognitive ageing: their unique brain integrity and adaptive traits challenge prevailing assumptions about ageing and highlight possible avenues for promoting cognitive health well into advanced life.

Further reading:

Eric Topol, *Super Agers: An Evidence-Based Approach to Longevity* (Simon & Schuster, 2025).

Julia Romano, *SuperAger: Insights into the Phenomenon of Successful Ageing* (2024).

David Cravit and Larry Wolf, *SuperAging: Getting Older Without Getting Old* (Flashpoint, 2023).Elise Marie Collins, *Super Ager: You Can Look Younger, Have More Energy, a Better Memory, and Live a Long and Healthy Life* (2018).

Peter Attia, *Outlive: The Science and Art of Longevity* (2023).

David A. Sinclair, *Lifespan: Why We Age – and Why We Don't Have To* (2019).

Aubrey de Grey and Michael Rae, *Ending Aging: The Rejuvenation Breakthroughs that Could Reverse Human Aging in Our Lifetime* (2007).

Ray Kurzweil and Terry Grossman, *Fantastic Voyage: Live Long Enough to Live Forever* (2004).

Elizabeth Blackburn and Elissa Epel, *The Telomere Effect: A Revolutionary Approach to Living Younger, Healthier, Longer* (2017).

About the Author

Suzanne Visser's life and work embody the essence of ikigai, a sense of purpose woven through presence, connection, and action. A legal scholar, publisher, and certified somatic practitioner, Suzanne brings a wealth of expertise to her coaching and consulting practice, Find Your iKiGAi, based in Central Australia. With over 25 years of experience in law, sustainability, and community leadership, she has guided high-performing executives, artists, and those recovering from burnout toward lives of balance and fulfilment. Her eleven years in Japan, during the vibrant economic bubble, shaped her understanding of ikigai as a lived practice. Influences such as her calligraphy teacher and the Body Weather Laboratory in Japan left a lasting imprint.

Fluent in five languages, Suzanne's global perspective is enriched by her extensive travels and her role as a sustainable justice expert and managing director of three successful businesses.

Visser has lived in Central Australia since 2000. She now writes in English. Visser is a versatile and productive writer of fiction and non-fiction.

Short stories: *De pracht van het dagelijks leven*; 1991, Bert Bakker (The Glory of Daily Life)

Thriller: *De Vismoorden*; Atlas Uitgeverij, 2000; published in German as *Das Japanische Rätsel*, DVA, 2001; in French as *Les Meurtres au Poisson*, Noir sur Blanc, 2002; in Spanish as *Sushi*, Ediciones B., 2003; in English as *The Fish Murders*, Clear Mind Press, 2022

Children's book: De Verdwijning, Leopold, 2005 (Vanishing)

Novel: *Terra Nostra*, Bookhost, 2003

Novel: *Een man met mooie benen*, Mistral, 2006 (A Bloke With Beautiful Legs

Non-fiction: *I, Unborn, Undying (a Search for the Self)*, For a Clear Mind, 2016

Non-fiction: *The Elephant's Tooth, Crime in Alice Springs*, Clear Mind Press 2022

The Elephant's Tooth, Crime in Rural Australia, Clear Mind Press 2022

Fiction, under pen name Shan: The Carpetbaggers of Mbantua, Clear Mind Press 2022

Non-fiction: *Marks on Paper, Essays on drawing, seeing and looking*, Clear Mind Press 2023

Fictional memoir, under pen name Shan: Women! 1. *Crying Mothers*

Women! 2. The Spirit of the Fox

Women! 3. Journey to the Edge, Clear Mind Press 2023

Non-fiction: *Never Retire, an exploration of old age*, Clear Mind Press 2023

Fiction: *Cash!* Clear Mind Press 2024

Poetry: *Hundred Fifty Five Sonnets*, Clear Mind Press 2025

Non-Fiction: *The Great Kitschification*, Clear Mind Press 2025

About this Book

What makes life worth living? Not in general, but specifically for you? In *Find Your ikigai*, Suzanne Visser guides you on a transformative trip to uncover your unique sense of meaning. Blending the wisdom of Japanese ikigai with Western insights of glow, flow and resilience, this book offers a gentle path toward healing and joy. Through eleven weeks of somatic practices, Suzanne helps you reconnect with your body, release stress, and rediscover your sense of meaning. Whether you're older or recovering from burnout, stress, illness or pain, this guide invites you to move from freeze to flow, one small step at a time.

Legal Page

Find Your iKiGAi

© Suzanne Visser

Published by Clear Mind Press, 2025, in Alice Springs, Australia

ISBN Print: 978-1-7641690-0-4

EISBN Ebook: 978-1-7641690-1-1

Typeset: Clear Mind Press

Cover design: Clear Mind Press

Portrait of the author: Hazel Blake

All inquiries should be made to the publisher: info@clearmindpress.com

https://www.clearmindpress.com

www.ingramcontent.com/pod-product-compliance
Lightning Source LLC
Chambersburg PA
CBHW051247020426
42333CB00025B/3099